Vert Maxx

Maximize Your Vertical – Reaching 6 to 12 More Inches

Fellow Jump Enthusiast and Friend,

Congratulations, if you're reading this then you have taken the first steps to reaching new heights in your sport – Getting the jump program!

Whether or not you have the digital version or the physical book in your hands you NOW have the resources you need to maximize your Vertical, enhance your Agility and Improve your overall Performance on and off the court or field.

If **You promise** me that you will stick to each week, each day, each exercise, each set, and each rep as outlined in the following pages then you will not be disappointed with your result. I **promise.**

TIP:
I noticed that while completing this program there were certain exercises that were easier than others for me to perform. If this happens for you I suggest pushing yourself a little bit. If the instruction is to perform 10 reps but you know you could 15 or 20 don't be afraid to take the liberty of adding a challenge for yourself. However, do not do less reps because its hard. If you find a certain exercise or set to be particularly hard take some extra rest time, massage your legs, and give it another go!

Keep me in the loop:
If you need a way to help you remain accountable to someone or you'd like your results to be published in the VM Newsletter please email me. Send your beginning vertical and your completion vertical along with any companion photos to emphasize your results.

info@vertmaxx.com

–Tim Howie

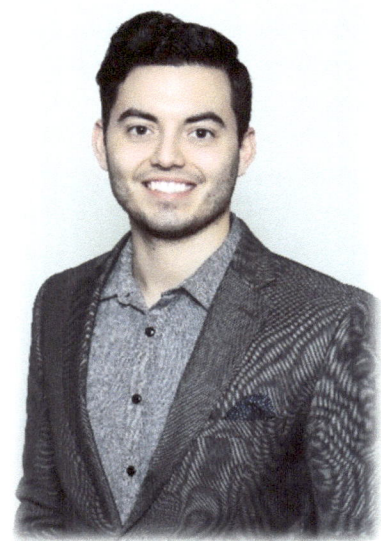

Table of Contents

Vert Maxx: Maximize your vertical
You get out what you put in!

It is with great pleasure that we present this program to you. To be frank your results are only guaranteed if you 1) Finish the program and 2) Push yourself during every set and every rep. Having said that, this program really works you will jump higher at the end of 15 weeks reaching the peak of your performance 30-45 days after completion – provided you remain active.

We are convinced that jumping enthusiasts will fall in love with our training program and will not need to look anywhere else.

As a jump enthusiast, it is of utmost importance to rely on cutting down your reaction time and teaching your body how to jump as quickly as possible, while jumping.

I have a lot of people ask me, "How many sets and reps should I do, Tim?" Now, I cannot specifically answer this question as every individual is different and has different goals.

When deciding on how many sets and reps to do, it begins with asking "What am I trying to get out of this workout?!"

This is where Vert Maxx comes into play. We changed the number of sets and reps, and, most importantly, we changed the number of days per week that the program will be completed compared to other programs on the market which will help with overall muscle recovery and strength development

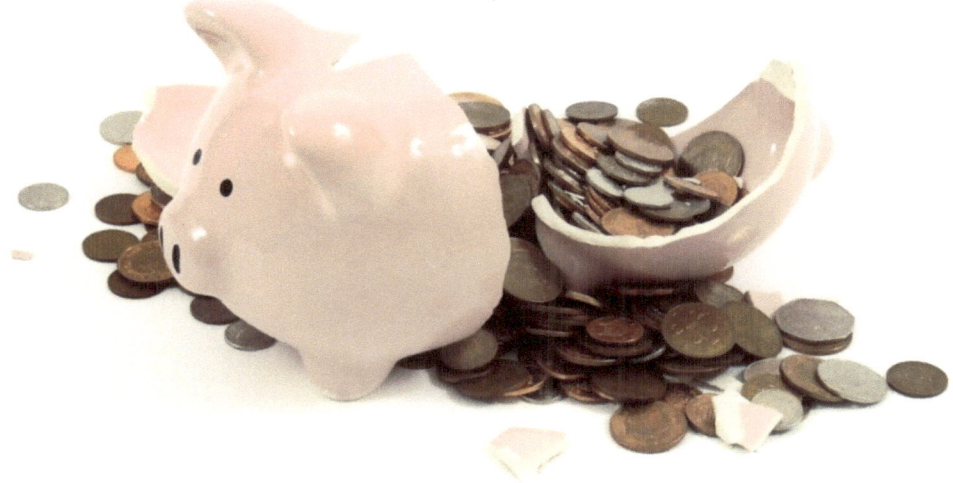

Why Vert Maxx is SO MUCH MORE than a jump program?

When you read or implement any exercise from the Vert Maxx Program the content MUST be read and followed as written.

a) Frequency- Vert Maxx is designed to be done 3 days per week, however you need to do it 4 times in week 15. This 3-day workout schedule alters each week to help you recover your muscle and strength of your legs because if you continue to follow a workout without any change, it can place you in a tough plateau to break. Aside from that, it can hinder your results and make your workouts tedious. This is extremely important in building the strength required for giving you the lift you need.

b) Log/Chart - Week 13 is designed as a complete muscle recovery week. It is very important that you follow your workout regime. With Vert Maxx, we have provided you with 2 workout charts at the back of this booklet.

Odd Numbered Week - Same order sequence for each exercise but actual days are different than in Even Numbered Weeks. [Monday-Wednesday-Friday]

Even Numbered Week - Same order sequence for each exercise but actual days are different than in Odd Numbered Weeks. [Tuesday-Wednesday-Thursday]

Great care must be taken to continually perform the workout programs as prescribed on the days designated in Vert Maxx for the respective week.

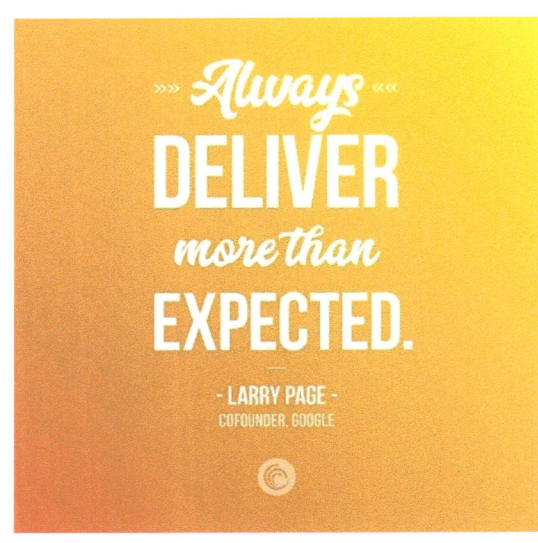

Week 13 - This week is designed for complete muscle recovery as it will allow the body time to repair and strengthen itself in preparation for week 15.

Please NOTE – Vert Maxx should not be completed at all during week 13.

Week 15 - This is the final week of the Vert Maxx Program. The workout planned and designed this week will completely break down the muscles, shock them and prepare them for the final recovery.

c) Repair and Recovery - Rest days are important, if you constantly break down muscle without a recovery period, you won't give the muscle fibers a chance to repair and build back stronger.

d) Resting Between Sets - The Vert Maxx workout consists of multiple sets and repetitions for each exercise. Here are some significant rules to follow for each of them: Once you complete SET 1 of an exercise it is NOT advisable to rest more than 2 minutes PRIOR to completing SET 2, then SET 3, etc.

In the workout environment, a common problem is muscle tenderness, soreness and pain. A new study shows that kneading or massaging muscles after hard exercise decreases inflammation and helps your muscles recover. So, it is important to massage the muscle during the 2-minute resting phase. AND remember to hydrate. If you are doing Stiff ups, be sure to massage your thighs while resting. When moving from an exercise to a new exercise (for example, from Stiff ups to Calf raises), do not rest at all. Move IMMEDIATELY to the next exercise without a rest period.

It is advised to rest 1-2 minutes in between all sets.

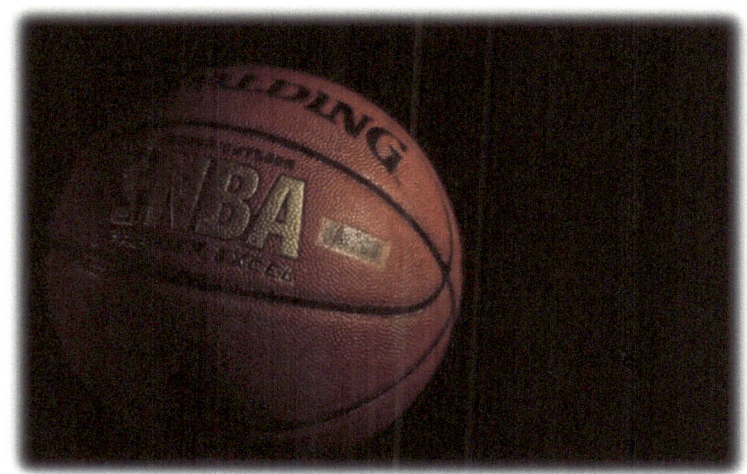

Vert Maxx Dynamic Stretching Warm-Up

5-8 Minutes

Knee Pulse to Full Extension (12 reps per side)
- ▶ On every 3rd or 5th jogging or walking step bring one knee up toward your chest while swinging the opposite arm around to meet your knee at its highest point. No contact needs to be made.
- ▶ Take another step and just before the 2nd step lift the same knee and swing the same opposing arm. This time, you are extending your leg fully into a high kick trying to touch your fingers to your toes
- ▶ This completes 2 reps for that leg
- ▶ You should feel this in your glutes and hamstrings

Calve Swings (12 reps per side)
- ▶ On every 3rd or 5th jogging or walking step extend one leg, keeping it straight, while resting on the heel
- ▶ Bend the opposite knee and sit slightly back to briefly stretch your straight leg
- ▶ Swing arms from straight back through to the front
- ▶ This completes one rep

Alternating Lateral Lunges (20 reps total)
- ▶ Have your left or right side facing the direction you wish to travel
- ▶ Extend leg for a wide stance and bend/lunge into the extended leg ensuring your knee and ankle are aligned
- ▶ This completes one rep
- ▶ Repeat with other leg
- ▶ Sitting up and bringing your opposite leg across your body, pivoting on your first foot
- ▶ Extending the other leg for another lunge

Bum Kicks (24-30 reps – 12-15/side)
- ▶ You're not going for distance, inch along until reps are completed
- ▶ Kick your heel up to your bum alternating sides after each kick
- ▶ Each bum kick completes one rep

High Knees (24-30 reps – 12-15/side)
- ▶ You're not going for distance, inch along until reps are completed
- ▶ Fire one knee up toward your chest, you should be stopping your legs when thighs are 90° and parallel to the floor
- ▶ This completes one rep
- ▶ Land on the balls of your feet rather than flat footed

Two Minute Skip or Run
- ▶ Moderate pace this is not a sprint
- ▶ Heart should be active not racing
- ▶ Not out of breath we are only warming up

VERT MAXX MAIN SET

Stiff Ups:

Starting Position & Movement:

▶ When beginning, bend down to a 1/4 squat position with your hands out in front of you and jump up.

▶ When jumping, keep your hands by your side or in front of you for assistance in jumping and follow the same procedures just described.

Mechanics:

Phase 1: Jump up into the air to a minimum of 8 to 10 inches. (You may jump 10 to 12 inches if this is too easy).

Phase 2: When in the air, your hands should be back by your side. When you land, this completes 1 repetition.

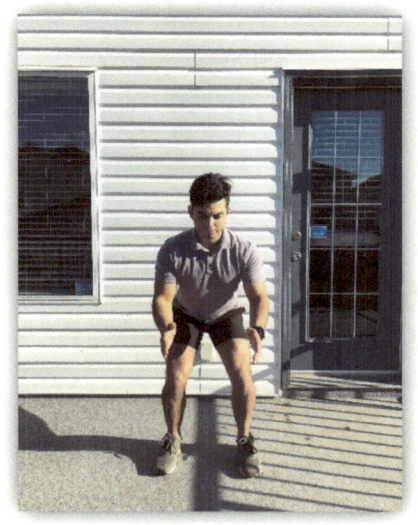 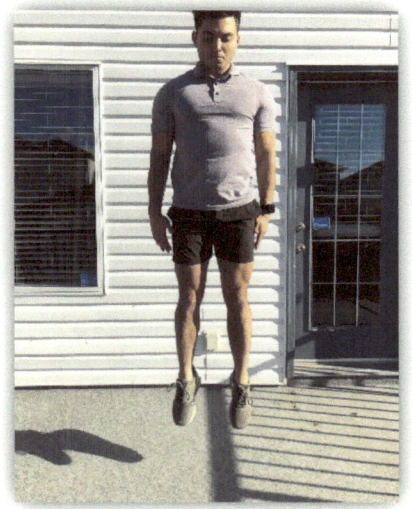

Notes

Calf Raises:

An easy exercise to do anywhere – you can knock out a set while brushing your teeth or waiting for the kettle to boil – and strong calves are essential to strong jumping activity.

Starting Position & Movement:

▶ Your starting position wi l be with the heel below the book or stair step rested on by your entire body.

▶ Stand up straight, then push through the balls of your feet and raise your heel until you are standing on your toes.

Mechanics:

Phase 1: Raise yourself as high up as you can with only the one calf.

Phase 2: Lower your body back to the original, starting position. This completes 1 repetition.

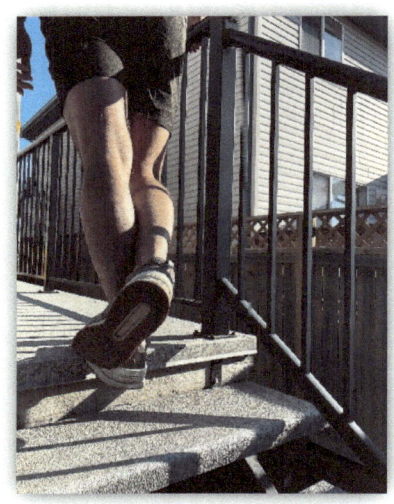 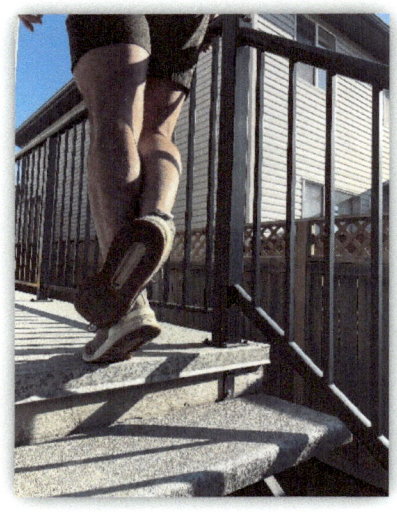

Notes:

Step Ups:

Step-ups hit all the major muscle groups in your lower body and will help your body burn more calories than usual during strength training sessions to shape your butt, perfectly!

Starting Position & Movement:

- ▶ Before you start, find a step, chair, or bench that when you place your foot on it, your knee bends to a 90-degree angle.

- ▶ Begin with one thigh on the chair parallel to the ground.

Mechanics:

Phase 1: With all of your strength, push off of the elevated leg and leap off of the chair as high as you can.

Phase 2: Crisscross or switch your legs in the air.

Phase 3: Land with the opposite leg elevated in the chair as in step 1. Repeat so that you are back to your starting leg. This completes 1 repetition.

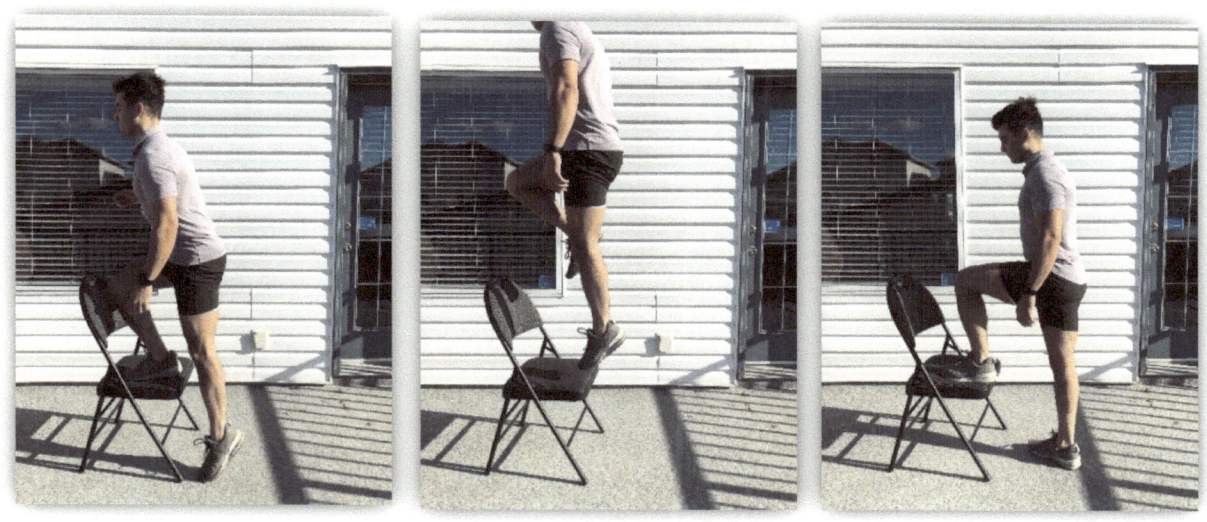

Notes:

Thrusts:

Thrusts is an exercise designed primarily to strengthen your calves and to strengthen the sides of your thighs and help with elasticity of the Achilles tendons. This exercise develops the muscles required for quick, repeating jumps.

Starting Position & Movement:

▶ Begin with heels slightly elevated

▶ With your legs straight.

Mechanics:

Phase 1: Simply jump straight up without bending your knees (It is helpful to use your arms to throw yourself into the air).

Phase 2: The split second you hit the ground, thrust back up as high as you can trying not to bend your legs. This completes 1 repetition.

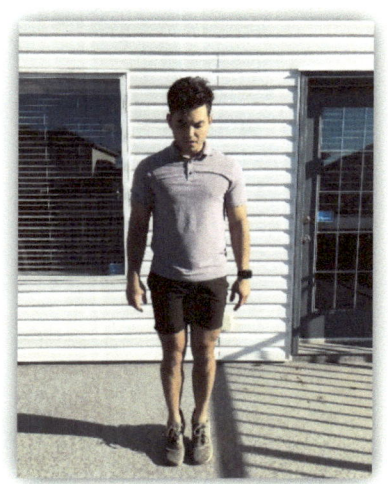 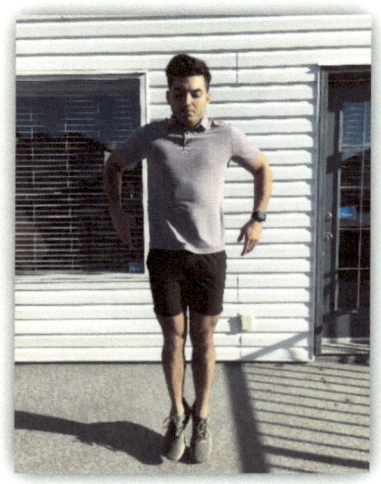

Notes:

Maxx Outs:

Max out your calves!

Starting Position & Movement:

▶ Stay elevated as high as possible on your tiptoes to assure that you work the high end of your calves.

Mechanics:

Phase 1: As quickly as you possibly can, jump repeatedly no more than 1/2 to 1 inch off the ground

Phase 2: Keep yourself elevated high on your tiptoes to ensure that you're working the upper calf muscles.

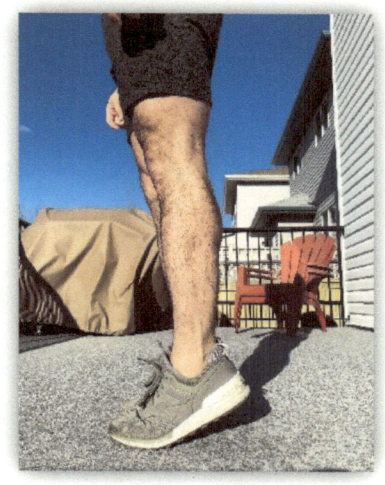 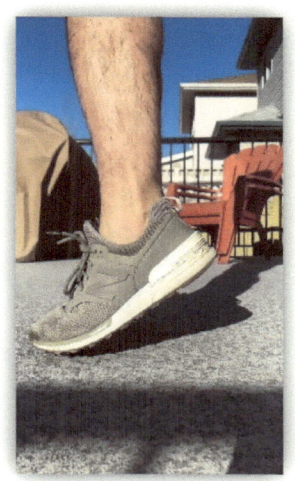

Notes:

VERT HOPS

Do you want well shaped thighs and legs? Vert hops help exercise the quads and calves while helping you tone your body as well.

Starting Position & Movement:

- ▶ For balance, hold a basketball or volleyball at chest level
- ▶ You can hold the ball with your hands at each side of the ball or hug the ball
- ▶ Squat down into a sitting position while holding the ball
- ▶ Make sure that you are looking straight ahead, with your back straight and that you are elevated on the balls of your feet (half tiptoed)
- ▶ Most importantly, make sure that your thighs are parallel to the ground.

Mechanics:

Phase 1: Hop or bounce in the seated position between 3-5 inches per hop. Keep your thighs parallel. When you land, that completes 1 repetition.

Phase 2: After you complete each repetition (each landing), you land back in the original, seated position. Jump up again for the next repetition.

Phase 3: At the completion (the last rep) of the required set, blast off as high as you possibly can. For example, if you are required to do 1 set of 15 repetitions, you will do 14 Vert Hops (3-5 inches per jump) and on the 15th Vert Hop, you will blast off as high as you possibly can.

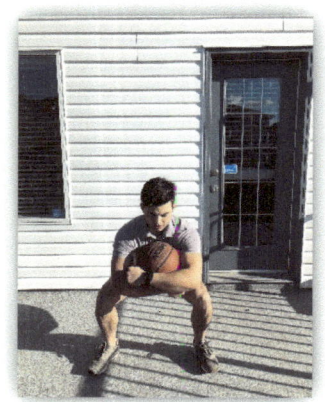 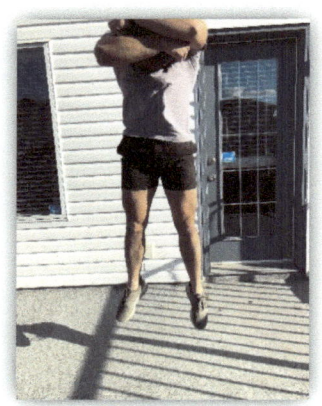

Notes:

Vert Maxx Cool Down / Stretching

10 Minutes

*Find a flat soft spot on the floor or with a mat and hold each stretch for 45-60 seconds

Single Leg Extension
- ▶ Extend one leg with toes pointing to the sky
- ▶ Bring opposite foot into inner thigh or as close as you can
- ▶ Reach for your toes or heel
- ▶ Bending at your hips not curling your back
- ▶ Hold when you feel a stretch
- ▶ Switch legs

Butterfly
- ▶ Bring heels together in front of you
- ▶ Hold feet together with your hands
- ▶ Bring heels toward your body until you feel a stretch
- ▶ Lean forward or pull heels closer to you for a deeper stretch

Modified Cross Legs
- ▶ Lay one leg in front of you heel and knee are straight across from each other
- ▶ Lay your opposite leg on top with your heel at the knee of the bottom leg and your top knee aligned with the bottom heel
- ▶ Compress top knee to bottom ankle for deeper stretch
- ▶ Compress and lean over legs for even deeper stretch
- ▶ Switch legs

Heel Seat
- ▶ Kneel on floor with good posture and toes pointed behind you (top of your foot resting on the ground)
- ▶ Sit back as far as you can (the goal being to sit on your heels)
- ▶ Place hands on ground on either side of you for needed support
- ▶ Stop where you feel the stretch

Standing Toe Touch
- ▶ Stand up straight
- ▶ Lean forward bending at the hips
- ▶ Reach with your hands as far down as you can (the goal being touching your toes or hands flat on the floor)

Standing Single Quad Stretch
- ▶ Standup straight
- ▶ Bend one knee bringing your heel towards your bum
- ▶ Hold onto the heel with that same side hand and keep hips level
- ▶ Be near a wall or other support if needed
- ▶ Switch legs

Vert Maxx Program Will:

1. Increase your vertical - respective to the effort you put into your training.

2. Help motivate you to jump aggressively when you play.

3. Maximize your jumping ability, peaking 30-45 days after completing the program.

4. Completely exhaust and breakdown the jumping muscles on the final week and prepare them for final recovery. That is why repetitions are higher, and 4 days are required instead of 3.

5. Maintain your new vertical by repeating week 8 on the alternating odd and even week routine or by aggressively playing a jumping sport 20-25 times per week.

If you wish to redo the program entirely for additional gains, you should wait at least 1 full month before restarting. It is important to rest your legs if you wish to add additional inches.

GET TO WORK AND
ENJOY REACHING NEW HEIGHTS!

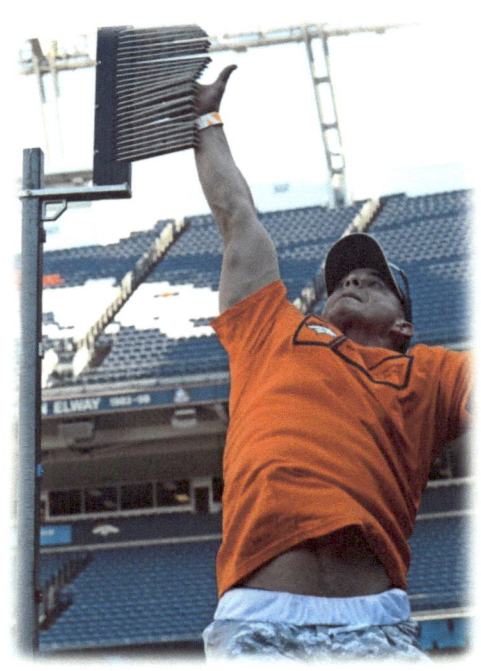

Some Mental and Emotional Benefits of Exercise

www.helpguide.org

Sharper memory and thinking.
The same endorphins that make you feel better also help you concentrate and feel mentally sharp for tasks at hand. Exercise also stimulates the growth of new brain cells and helps prevent age-related decline.

Higher self-esteem.
Regular activity is an investment in your mind, body, and soul. When it becomes habit, it can foster your sense of self-worth and make you feel strong and powerful. You'll feel better about your appearance and, by meeting even small exercise goals, you'll feel a sense of achievement.

Better sleep.
Even short bursts of exercise in the morning or afternoon can help regulate your sleep patterns. If you prefer to exercise at night, relaxing exercises such as yoga or gentle stretching can help promote sleep.

More energy.
Increasing your heart rate several times a week will give you more get-up-and-go. Start off with just a few minutes of exercise per day and increase your workout as you feel more energized.

Stronger resilience.
When faced with mental or emotional challenges in life, exercise can help you cope in a healthy way, instead of resorting to alcohol, drugs, or other negative behaviors that ultimately only make your symptoms worse. Regular exercise can also help boost your immune system and reduce the impact of stress.

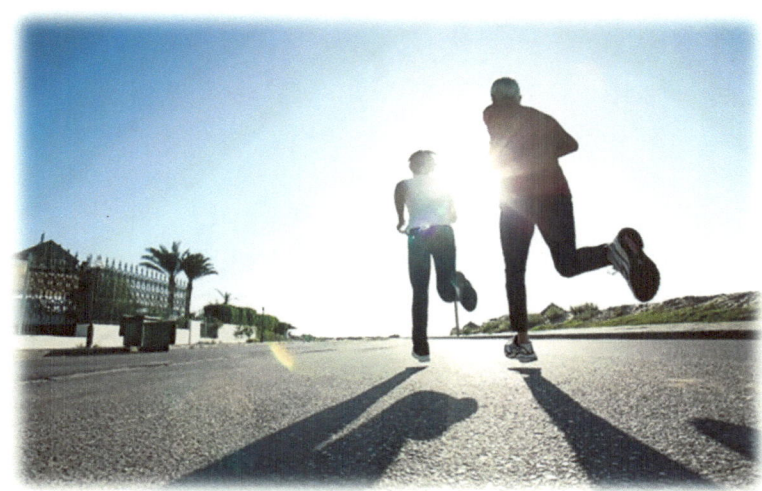

Staying Motivated with Mental Health Struggles

www.helpguide.org

Focus on activities you enjoy.

Any activity that gets you moving counts. That could include throwing a Frisbee with a dog or friend, walking laps of a mall window shopping, or cycling to the grocery store. If you've never exercised before or don't know what you might enjoy, try a few different things. Activities such as gardening or tackling a home improvement project can be great ways to start moving more when you have a mood disorder—as well as helping you become more active, they can also leave you with a sense of purpose and accomplishment.

Be comfortable.

Whatever time of day you decide to exercise, wear clothing that's comfortable and choose a setting that you find calming or energizing. That may be a quiet corner of your home, a scenic path, or your favorite city park.

Reward yourself.

Part of the reward of completing an activity is how much better you'll feel afterwards, but it always helps your motivation to promise yourself an extra treat for exercising. Reward yourself with a hot bubble bath after a workout, a delicious smoothie, or with an extra episode of your favorite TV show.

Make exercise a social activity.

Exercising with a friend or loved one, or even your kids, will not only make exercising more fun and enjoyable, it can also help motivate you to stick to a workout routine. You'll also feel better than if you were exercising alone. In fact, when you're suffering from a mood disorder such as depression, the companionship can be just as important as the exercise.

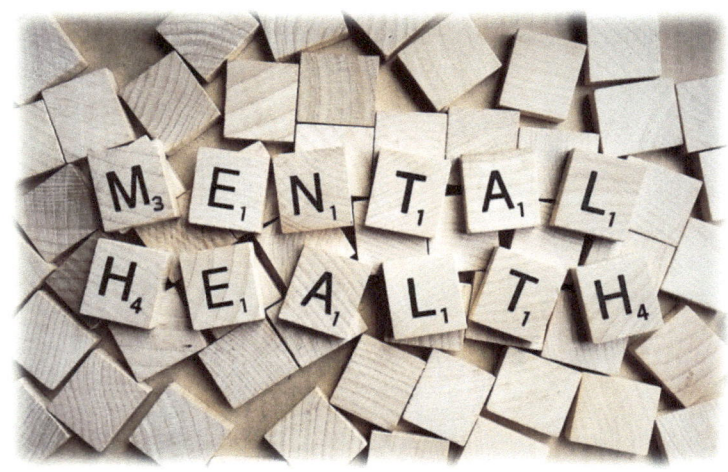

Stretching: Focus on Flexibility

www.mayoclinic.org

Stretching may take a back seat to your exercise routine. The main concern is exercising, not stretching, right?

Not so fast. Stretching may help you:

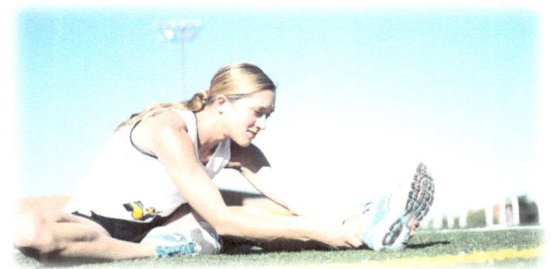

- ▶ Improve your joint range of motion
- ▶ Improve your athletic performance
- ▶ Decrease your risk of injury

Understand why stretching can help and how to stretch correctly.

Benefits of stretching

Studies about the benefits of stretching have had mixed results. Some show that stretching helps. Other studies show that stretching before or after exercise has little to no benefit.

Some research shows that stretching doesn't reduce muscle soreness after exercise, and other studies show that static stretching performed immediately before a sprint event may slightly worsen performance.

Stretching can help improve flexibility, and, consequently, range of motion about your joints. Better flexibility may:

- ▶ Improve your performance in physical activities
- ▶ Decrease your risk of injuries
- ▶ Help your joints move through their full range of motion
- ▶ Enable your muscles to work most effectively

Stretching also increases blood flow to the muscle. You may learn to enjoy the ritual of stretching before or after hitting the trail, ballet floor or soccer field.

Stretching essentials

Before you plunge into stretching, make sure you do it safely and effectively. While you can stretch anytime, anywhere, be sure to use proper technique. Stretching incorrectly can actually do more harm than good.

Use these tips to keep stretching safe:

► **Don't consider stretching a warmup.** You may hurt yourself if you stretch cold muscles. Before stretching, warm up with light walking, jogging or biking at low intensity for five to 10 minutes. Even better, stretch after your workout when your muscles are warm.

Consider skipping stretching before an intense activity, such as sprinting or track and field activities. Some research suggests that pre-event stretching may actually decrease performance. Research has also shown that stretching immediately before an event weakens hamstring strength.

Instead of static stretching, try performing a "dynamic warmup." A dynamic warm-up involves performing movements similar to those in your sport or physical activity at a low level, then gradually increasing the speed and intensity as you warm up.

► **Strive for symmetry.** Everyone's genetics for flexibility are a bit different. Rather than striving for the flexibility of a dancer or gymnast, focus on having equal flexibility side to side (especially if you have a history of a previous injury). Flexibility that is not equal on both sides may be a risk factor for injury.

► **Focus on major muscle groups.** Concentrate your stretches on major muscle groups such as your calves, thighs, hips, lower back, neck and shoulders. Make sure that you stretch both sides.

Also stretch muscles and joints that you routinely use.

► **Don't bounce.** Stretch in a smooth movement, without bouncing. Bouncing as you stretch can injure your muscle and actually contribute to muscle tightness.

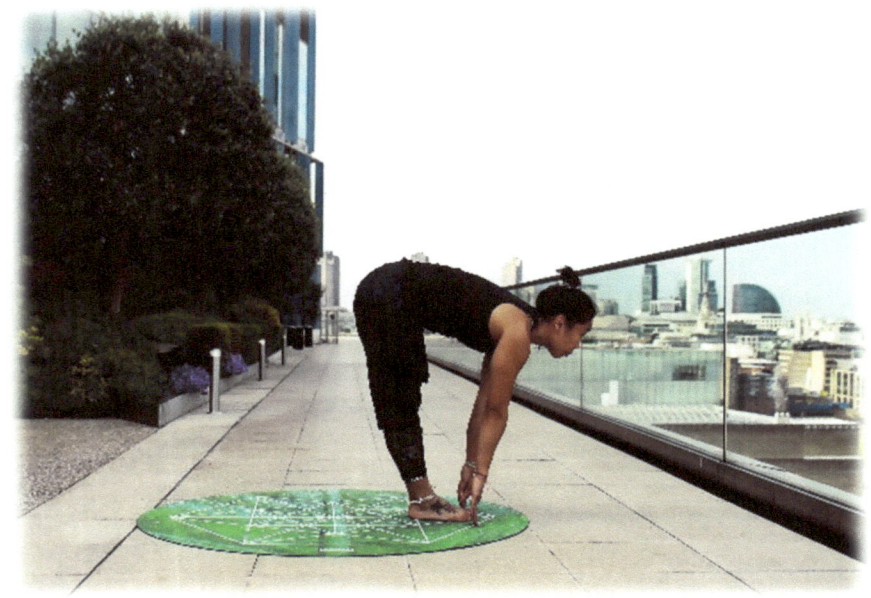

▶ **Hold your stretch.** Breathe normally and hold each stretch for about 30 seconds; in problem areas, you may need to hold for around 60 seconds.

▶ **Don't aim for pain.** Expect to feel tension while you're stretching, not pain. If it hurts, you've pushed too far. Back off to the point where you don't feel any pain, then hold the stretch.

▶ **Make stretches sport specific.** Some evidence suggests that it's helpful to do stretches involving the muscles used most in your sport or activity. If you play soccer, for instance, stretch your hamstrings as you're more vulnerable to hamstring strains. So, opt for stretches that help your hamstrings.

▶ **Keep up with your stretching.** Stretching can be time-consuming. But you can achieve the most benefits by stretching regularly, at least two to three times a week.

▶ **Bring movement into your stretching.** Gentle movements, such as those in tai chi or yoga, can help you be more flexible in specific movements. These types of exercises can also help reduce falls in seniors.

▶ Remember the "dynamic warmup:" If you're going to perform a specific activity, such as a kick in martial arts or kicking a soccer ball, start out slowly and at low intensity to get your muscles used to it. Then speed up gradually.

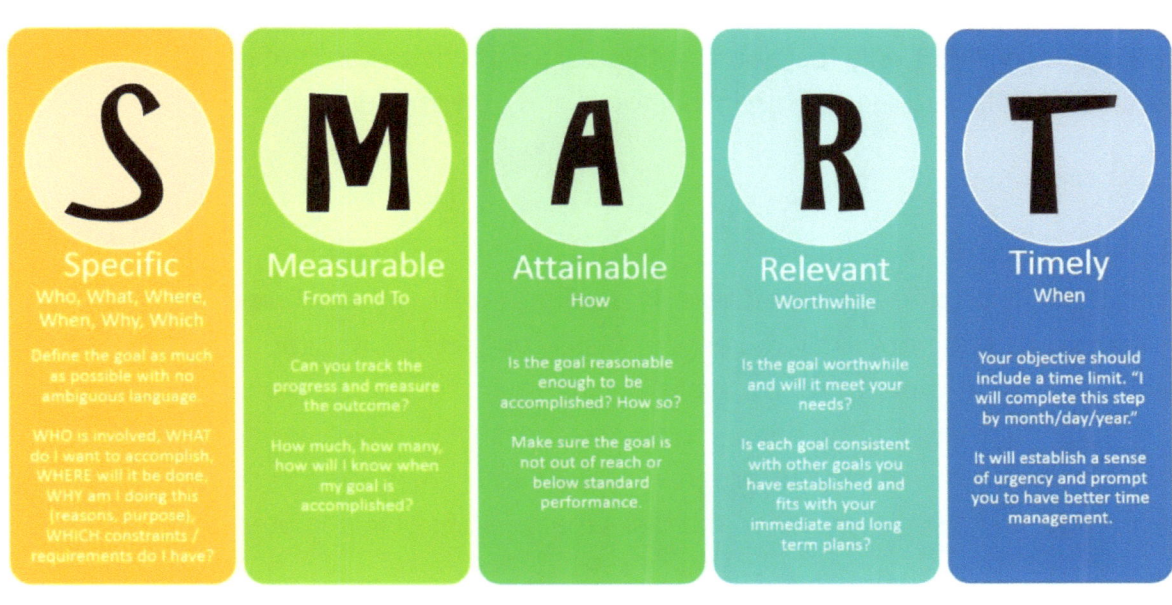

Four Ways to Track Your Progress Towards Your Goals

Tiffany Mason – www.lifehack.org

1. Look at the big picture

This is the foundation of keeping track of your progress and also accomplishing your goals. A lot of us just go through the motions day-to-day. We are on pure "survival mode" rather than living each day to its fullest. In order for you to start tracking your progress, you must take a step back and look at the big picture. Why do you do what you do? What is the purpose of waking up in the morning and getting the day started? Think about these things and answer these questions with the end result in mind. Where do you see yourself in the future in every aspect of your life? Take the time to reflect upon your goals and imagine what the big picture looks like. It's important for you to see the bigger picture rather than just living day-to-day with no direction or motivation.

2. Plan and Organize

When it comes to tracking your progress toward your goals, planning and organizing your time is key to accomplishing your goals. Once you are clear with the big picture, you must now plan and organize the necessary steps that you need to take in order to accomplish your goals. Take your calendar and plan on organizing your time around achieving all your goals. Having a planner or using your iPhone or Google calendar is a great way to track your progress. Each week you will have specific goals that you want to accomplish. Throughout each week, you will have a To-Do list that you will work on every day. When you are able to plan and organize your time wisely, you will not only feel good that you are working toward your goals but you are also developing life skills such as self discipline, focus and determination.

3. Accountability

Share your goals with your spouse or a good friend. It's important to have another person ask you about your progress. When there is someone else other than yourself holding you accountable, you are more likely to get your tasks completed throughout the week. You will be motivated by both the desire to avoid letting them down as well as the support and encouragement that they offer when you do accomplish your goals. Working with a life coach is a great way to help you track your progress toward your goals. When I share my goals with my husband, it helps me stay focused on the tasks that need to be completed.

4. Celebrate

With each accomplishment, it's important for you to take a step back and celebrate your success. If you are constantly looking ahead and never taking the time to celebrate your accomplishments, you will most likely get burnt out. When you get burnt out, you lose the motivation to stay focused on your goals. I know that I am guilty of constantly looking ahead and focusing on the next big thing. What has really helped me stay motivated in accomplishing my goals is celebrating along the way. Celebrating your accomplishments is a way for you to track your progress toward your goals because you are able to stop and appreciate your hard work before moving onto your next goal. Whenever you accomplish a goal, make sure you take the time to celebrate.

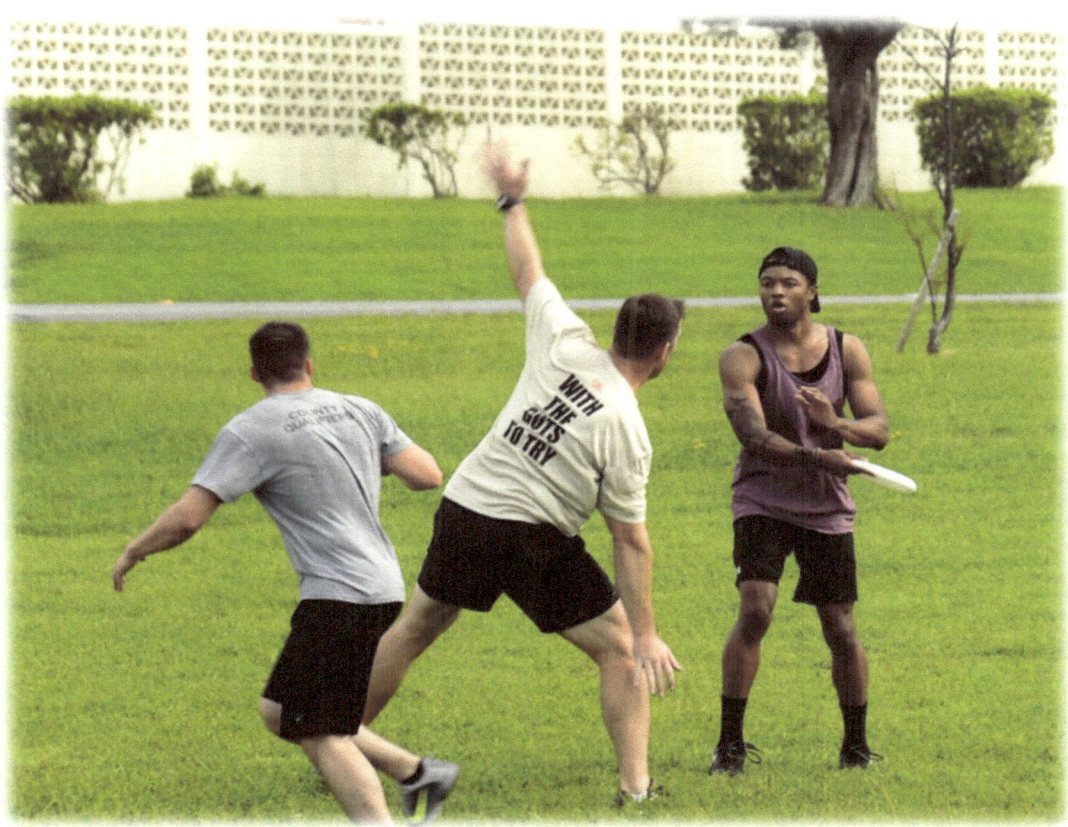

Vert Maxx Log (Odd Weeks)

Mon - Wed - Fri

W	Stiff Ups		Calf Raises		Step Ups		Thrusts		Maxx Outs		Vert Hops	
	Sets	Reps	Sets	Reps	Sets	Reps	Sets	Reps	Sets	Reps	Sets	Reps
1	2	20	2	10	2	10	2	15	1	100	4	15
Track												
3	3	25	2	20	2	15	2	25	1	300	4	20
Track												
5	4	25	2	30	2	20	2	35	2	250	4	25
Track												
7	4	30	2	40	2	25	2	50	2	350	5	25
Track												
9	4	50	2	50	2	30	2	70	3	300	5	30
Track												
11	6	50	4	30	2	35	2	90	4	275	5	30
Track												
13	**DO NOT PERFORM VERT MAXX THIS WEEK - REST YOUR LEGS**											
15*	4	100	4	50	2	50	2	100	4	500	5	50
Track												

* Week 15 to be completed on Monday-Tuesday-Thursday-Friday.

Vert Maxx Log (Even Weeks)

Tue - Wed - Thur

W	Stiff Ups		Calf Raises		Step Ups		Thrusts		Maxx Outs		Vert Hops	
	Sets	Reps	Sets	Reps	Sets	Reps	Sets	Reps	Sets	Reps	Sets	Reps
2	3	20	2	15	2	15	2	20	1	200	4	20
Track												
4	3	30	2	25	2	20	2	30	2	200	4	20
Track												
6	2	50	2	35	2	25	2	40	2	300	4	30
Track												
8	3	50	2	45	2	30	2	60	4	200	5	25
Track												
10	5	40	2	55	2	35	2	80	4	250	5	30
Track												
12	4	75	4	35	2	40	2	100	4	300	6	30
Track												
14*	3	30	2	30	2	20	2	30	1	250	4	20
Track												

* Week 14 is preparing your legs for Week 15. There is a reason behind this - don't get cocky!